COMPLETE GUIDE TO CELIAC DISEASE

A Comprehensive Handbook For Understanding, Managing, And Thriving With Gluten Sensitivity Expert Guidance, Recipes, And Lifestyle Strategies For Holistic Wellness

DEHART HAIRSTON

DISCLAIMER

This book's content is only intended for general informative purposes. At the time of writing, the author has taken every precaution to guarantee that the material is correct and current. Nevertheless, the author disclaims all explicit and implicit representations and guarantees about the availability, appropriateness, correctness, completeness, and usefulness of the material on these pages.

Since the author is not a licensed medical practitioner, the material in this book shouldn't be interpreted as medical advice. Before making any modifications to their diet, exercise regimen, or medical treatment, readers are urged to speak with a licensed healthcare provider.

Moreover, the author has no connection to any of the businesses, organizations, or people that are discussed in this book. Any mentions of goods, services, businesses, or people are purely informative and do not indicate endorsement or suggestion.

This book's content is entirely dependent on the author's expertise, study, and comprehension of the topic. Despite having taken reasonable care to offer correct information, the author disclaims all liability for any mistakes or omissions in the material as well as for any losses, harm, or damages resulting from using the information.

It is recommended that readers use their own judgment and discretion when applying the knowledge in this book to their own situations. The use or implementation of any material in this book may result in unfavorable repercussions, directly or indirectly, for which the author assumes no liability.

By reading this book, you agree to release and hold the author harmless from any claims, losses, liabilities, costs, or expenditures resulting from or related to the use of the information you get from it.

Table of Contents

CHAPTER 1 13

Understanding Celiac Disease......................13

What Is Celiac Disease?.................................13

Causes And Risk Factors..............................14

Common Symptoms.......................................15

CHAPTER 2 17

Diagnosis 17

How Is Celiac Disease Diagnosed?...............17

Blood Tests And Biopsy Procedures.............17

Understanding Test Results 18

CHAPTER 3 21

Gluten And Its Impact...................................21

What Is Gluten? 21

Gluten-Containing Foods 22

1. Bread and Pasta:....................................22

2. Processed Foods:...................................22

3. Beer and ale:...22

4. Cereals & Grains:..................................23

8. Desserts and sweets:.............................23

Effects Of Gluten On Celiac Patients....................24

2. Malabsorption: 24

3. Weariness and Weakness: 24

4. Skin Problems: 24

CHAPTER 4 27

Gluten-Free Diet Basics 27

Introduction To Gluten-Free Eating 27

Foods To Avoid And Foods To Enjoy 28

Tips For Grocery Shopping And Dining Out 30

CHAPTER 5 33

Managing Celiac Disease 33

Importance Of Strict Adherence To A Gluten-Free Diet 33

Dealing With Cross-Contamination 35

Lifestyle Adjustments For Better Health 37

CHAPTER 6 41

Living With Celiac Disease 41

Coping Strategies For Emotional And Social Challenges 41

Support Systems And Resources Available 44

Thriving Beyond The Diagnosis 47

CHAPTER 7 51

Gluten-Free Cooking And Recipes 51

Cooking Techniques And Ingredient Substitutions 51

  1. Grain Alternatives: 51

  2. Thickening Agents: 52

  3. Baking Tip: 52

  4. Cross-contamination Awareness: 52

  1. Flour Substitutes: 53

  2. Breadcrumbs: 53

  3. Soy Sauce Alternatives: 53

  4. Pasta Swaps: 53

Delicious Gluten-Free Recipes For Every Meal 54

  Breakfast: Gluten-free Banana Pancakes...........54

  Lunch: Quinoa salad with avocado and chickpeas. 55

  Dinner: Gluten-free Chicken Stir-Fry. 55

  Snack: Homemade trail mix........................56

Tips For Meal Planning And Batch Cooking 56

  1. Create a Weekly Menu:...........................56

  1. Label Containers:..................................57

  2. Use Reusable Containers:........................58

  3. Rotate Stock: 58

CHAPTER 8 59

Navigating Social Situations..59

Explaining Celiac Disease To Family And Friends59

Handling Social Events And Gatherings..................60

Advocating For Yourself In Various Settings 62

CHAPTER 9 65

Celiac Disease In Children 65

Recognizing Symptoms In Children......................65

Managing Celiac Disease In School Settings 66

Supporting Children With Celiac Disease 67

CHAPTER 10 69

Future Perspectives And Research........................69

Promising Advances In Celiac Disease Research...69

Potential Therapies And Treatments On The Horizon..72

Advocacy And Awareness Efforts For Celiac Disease 75

CONCLUSION...78

THE END 81

ABOUT THIS BOOK

This book, "Celiac Disease," is an essential resource for anybody afflicted by or interested in understanding this ailment. Celiac disease is a severe autoimmune illness caused by gluten ingestion that damages the small intestine. Chapter 1 of this book provides a complete introduction to celiac disease, including its etiology and prevalent symptoms. Understanding these fundamentals is critical for anybody dealing with unexplained health problems or looking to help loved ones with the disease.

Chapter 2 goes into the essential component of diagnosis, including the many tests and methods used to diagnose celiac disease. With simple explanations of blood testing, biopsy procedures, and how to interpret test findings, readers gain insight into the diagnostic process, allowing them to successfully advocate for their health.

Adopting a gluten-free diet is one of the most important parts of celiac disease management, as discussed in Chapter 4. This section offers practical advice on adjusting to gluten-free eating, finding foods to avoid and love, and confidently navigating grocery shopping and dining out. Adhering carefully to a gluten-free diet is critical for treating symptoms and avoiding complications, making this chapter required reading for celiac disease patients.

Beyond dietary issues, Chapter 5 of this book discusses the larger problems of living with celiac disease, highlighting the necessity of lifestyle changes and coping methods for emotional and social obstacles. This comprehensive approach continues in Chapter 6, which provides readers with coping skills, support networks, and tools for flourishing after the diagnosis, building resilience, and empowerment.

Furthermore, this book acknowledges the special obstacles that children with celiac disease experience, giving an entire chapter to understanding and treating the illness in school settings, as well as offering support to young patients and their families. Furthermore, in Chapter 10, this book looks forward, evaluating prospective scientific developments and arguing for better awareness and support for celiac disease patients.

With its complete discussion of diagnosis, treatment, lifestyle changes, and future views, "Celiac Disease" is more than simply a book; it's a lifeline for those dealing with an autoimmune condition. This book is a helpful companion on the path to greater health and well-being, whether you are newly diagnosed, supporting a loved one, or just want to enhance your knowledge.

CHAPTER 1

Understanding Celiac Disease

What Is Celiac Disease?

Celiac disease is a chronic autoimmune illness caused by consuming gluten, a protein present in wheat, barley, and rye. When a person with celiac disease consumes gluten, their immune system responds by destroying the lining of the small intestine. This damage hinders vitamin absorption from the diet, causing a variety of issues.

Imagine your small intestine as a carpet with tiny, finger-like projections known as villi. These villi aid in the digestion and absorption of nutrients. Gluten serves as a bully in celiac disease, inducing inflammation and flattening of the villi, limiting the available surface area for nutritional absorption. As a result, vital nutrients such as vitamins, minerals, and lipids are not effectively absorbed, resulting in long-term malnutrition.

Causes And Risk Factors

The actual etiology of celiac disease is unclear, however it is thought to be a mix of hereditary and environmental factors. People who have a family history of celiac disease are more likely to develop the ailment because specific genetic markers are related to it. Furthermore, environmental variables such as when gluten is introduced into an infant's diet and certain illnesses may contribute to the disease's onset.

Some people may have a genetic susceptibility to celiac disease but may not acquire it until provoked by an environmental condition such as a stressful event, surgery, pregnancy, or delivery. It is crucial to understand that celiac disease may occur at any age, from infancy to late adulthood.

Common Symptoms

Celiac disease symptoms may vary greatly between people, making it difficult to identify. While some individuals suffer digestive problems, others may exhibit non-digestive symptoms or be completely asymptomatic.

Chronic diarrhea, stomach discomfort, bloating, gas, and constipation are all possible digestive symptoms. However, other people may have no gastrointestinal problems at all. Instead, individuals may exhibit non-digestive symptoms such as weariness, anemia, joint discomfort, osteoporosis, dermatitis herpetiformis (a skin rash), or neurological symptoms such as headaches and peripheral neuropathy.

These many symptoms might make it difficult to identify celiac disease, causing delays in diagnosis and treatment.

As a consequence, patients may experience vitamin deficits and long-term problems before getting an accurate diagnosis.

Understanding these symptoms is critical since early discovery and treatment may prevent additional damage to the small intestine, improving overall health and quality of life in celiac disease patients. If you believe you or someone you know has celiac disease, you should see a doctor for an accurate diagnosis.

CHAPTER 2

Diagnosis

How Is Celiac Disease Diagnosed?

Celiac disease diagnosis requires a set of measures to effectively diagnose the ailment. Because celiac disease overlaps symptoms with other gastrointestinal illnesses, an accurate diagnosis is critical for successful treatment. Physicians usually start with a comprehensive medical history and physical exam, paying special attention to symptoms such as persistent diarrhea, stomach discomfort, weight loss, and exhaustion.

Blood Tests And Biopsy Procedures

Celiac disease is diagnosed mostly via blood testing. The principal blood test detects levels of particular antibodies that the body develops in response to gluten ingestion.

These antibodies, such as anti-tissue transglutaminase (tTG) and anti-endomysial antibodies (EMA), may suggest an immunological response to gluten. If these antibodies are high, it indicates the likelihood of celiac disease, necessitating additional testing.

In addition to blood testing, an endoscopy and biopsy are often used to confirm the diagnosis. An endoscopy involves inserting a thin, flexible tube with a camera via the mouth and into the small intestine. A tiny tissue sample (biopsy) is then extracted from the lining of the small intestine. This sample is evaluated under a microscope for celiac disease-related alterations, such as villous atrophy and increased intraepithelial lymphocytes.

Understanding Test Results

Interpreting celiac disease test results takes skill and consideration of several variables.

Elevated levels of celiac-specific antibodies in blood testing, together with typical abnormalities in intestinal biopsies, are significant indicators of celiac disease. However, it is critical to recognize that false-negative findings might occur, particularly if gluten has been removed from the diet before testing.

Furthermore, some people may have non-celiac gluten sensitivity, which may cause comparable symptoms but does not include the immune system reaction found in celiac disease. Proper interpretation of test data, together with clinical judgment, enables healthcare practitioners to establish accurate diagnoses and design suitable treatment strategies.

CHAPTER 3

Gluten And Its Impact

What Is Gluten?

Gluten is a protein present in wheat, barley, rye, and derivatives. It is what gives dough its elasticity and allows baked items to keep their form. This harmless protein, however, may hurt the health of those who have celiac disease.

Gluten is generally safe for most individuals in its natural condition. However, for people with celiac disease, even a modest quantity might cause an immunological reaction that destroys the small intestine. This might result in a variety of symptoms, ranging from gastrointestinal discomfort to starvation.

Gluten-Containing Foods

Identifying gluten-containing foods is critical for celiac disease patients to follow a gluten-free diet. While it may seem simple to avoid obvious sources such as bread and pasta, gluten may lurk in many unexpected areas.

Gluten is often found in the following foods:

1. Bread and Pasta: Traditional wheat-based bread, pasta, and baked items are high in gluten.

2. Processed Foods: Gluten is often disguised in processed foods as an ingredient or thickening. This includes soups, sauces, salad dressings, and processed meats.

3. Beer and ale: Most beers are made from barley, which includes gluten. Even some "gluten-free" beers may still contain gluten.

4. Cereals & Grains: While oats are gluten-free, they are often processed in facilities that also handle wheat, which may lead to cross-contamination. Furthermore, wheat-based cereals are frequent morning mainstays that contain gluten.

5. Gluten is often found in snack foods such as pretzels, crackers, and some kinds of chips.

6. Soy sauce, hoisin sauce, and other condiments may use gluten as a thickening agent.

7. Processed meats, such as sausages and deli meats, may include gluten as fillers or binders.

8. Desserts and sweets: Many desserts, such as cakes, cookies, pastries, and ice cream, contain gluten unless they are labeled gluten-free.

Effects Of Gluten On Celiac Patients

Consuming gluten may trigger a variety of symptoms and long-term health consequences in those with celiac disease. These effects vary greatly from person to person, but often include:

1. Symptoms of the gastrointestinal system include stomach discomfort, bloating, diarrhea, constipation, and nausea.

2. **Malabsorption:** Damage to the small intestine impairs the body's capacity to absorb nutrients, resulting in vitamin and mineral shortages.

3. **Weariness and Weakness:** Malnutrition due to malabsorption may cause weariness, weakness, and anemia.

4. **Skin Problems:** Some people with celiac disease may develop dermatitis herpetiformis, which is an itchy skin rash.

5. Celiac disease may sometimes produce neurological symptoms such as headaches, peripheral neuropathy, and seizures.

6. Celiac disease may cause joint discomfort and inflammation.

7. In children, undiagnosed or untreated celiac disease may cause delayed growth and development.

Individuals with celiac disease must rigorously follow a gluten-free diet to avoid these symptoms and limit the risk of long-term problems. Individuals with celiac disease may take control of their diet and enhance their general well-being by learning about gluten, identifying gluten-containing foods, and understanding the consequences of gluten on their health.

CHAPTER 4

Gluten-Free Diet Basics

Introduction To Gluten-Free Eating

Transitioning to a gluten-free diet might be scary at first, but with the correct information and tools, it becomes a lot easier. A gluten-free diet avoids foods containing gluten, a protein present in wheat, barley, rye, and, in certain cases, oats. Consuming gluten may cause an immunological reaction that damages the small intestine in those with celiac disease, resulting in a variety of health concerns.

Understanding which foods contain gluten is key. While obvious sources of gluten include bread, pasta, and baked products, it may also be found in sauces, spices, and processed meals. Reading ingredient labels becomes second nature for those following a gluten-free diet.

However, avoiding gluten does not imply compromising flavor or nutrients. Naturally, gluten-free foods include fruits, vegetables, lean meats, seafood, dairy products, legumes, nuts, and gluten-free grains such as rice, quinoa, and buckwheat. Individuals who embrace these entire foods may eat a broad and healthy diet while avoiding gluten-containing goods.

Foods To Avoid And Foods To Enjoy

To successfully follow a gluten-free diet, you must first learn which foods to avoid and which to embrace. Gluten may be found in a variety of commonly consumed foods, thus caution is advised.

Avoid foods that include wheat, barley, rye, or their derivatives. This includes bread, spaghetti, cereals, cakes, cookies, pastries, and beer, among other things.

Additionally, certain manufactured goods may have hidden gluten in the form of chemicals or flavorings, thus it is critical to carefully read labels.

On the other hand, a gluten-free diet provides a variety of tasty and healthy alternatives. Fresh fruits and vegetables are inherently gluten-free and include plenty of vitamins, minerals, and fiber. Lean proteins such as chicken, fish, eggs, and tofu, as well as dairy products such as milk, yogurt, and cheese, are all good options.

Gluten-free grains such as rice, maize, quinoa, and oats (certified gluten-free) may be palatable alternatives for gluten-containing foods. There is also a wide range of gluten-free flours and baking mixes available for folks who like baking.

Tips For Grocery Shopping And Dining Out

Navigating grocery store aisles and eating out while following a gluten-free diet needs some preparation and understanding.

When grocery shopping, begin by becoming acquainted with gluten-free brands and products. Many retailers now have separate gluten-free areas or prominently identify gluten-free foods throughout their stores. However, ingredients might vary, so always double-check the labels.

Choose naturally gluten-free foods wherever feasible, such as fresh vegetables, meat, poultry, fish, eggs, and dairy. When choosing packaged or processed goods, seek certified gluten-free labeling to verify they adhere to rigorous gluten-free guidelines.

When eating out, communication is essential. Inform your waitress of your dietary limitations, and inquire about gluten-free items on the menu. Many restaurants now provide gluten-free menus and may fulfill specific needs. Be wary of cross-contamination, particularly in kitchens that handle gluten-containing foods. It's OK to inquire about preparation procedures to guarantee your food stays gluten-free.

Consider trying ethnic cuisines like Mexican, Thai, or Japanese, which often have naturally gluten-free foods. Dining out may be pleasant without jeopardizing your dietary requirements with a little study and discussion.

Individuals with celiac disease may live a long and full life while reducing their risk of gluten-related health issues by learning the fundamentals of gluten-free nutrition. Managing a gluten-free diet becomes second nature with awareness, preparation, and a willingness to try new foods and dining alternatives.

CHAPTER 5

Managing Celiac Disease

Importance Of Strict Adherence To A Gluten-Free Diet

Living with celiac disease requires a lifetime commitment to a rigorous gluten-free diet. Why is this adherence so important? Let's get into it.

Gluten, a protein present in wheat, barley, and rye, causes an immunological reaction in people with celiac disease, destroying the lining of the small intestine. This damage may cause a variety of symptoms, including gastrointestinal disorders like bloating and diarrhea, as well as more systemic concerns like exhaustion and vitamin deficits. By removing gluten from your diet, you may stop the damage and enable your gut to repair.

The problem, however, is that gluten is so widely distributed. It may lurk in unexpected areas, including sauces, soups, cosmetics, and pharmaceuticals. This highlights the necessity of reading labels carefully and being aware of possible sources of gluten contamination.

Furthermore, strictly adhering to a gluten-free diet is more than simply treating symptoms; it is also about avoiding long-term consequences. Untreated celiac disease may lead to major complications such as osteoporosis, infertility, and some forms of cancer. Individuals with celiac disease who avoid gluten may greatly lower their risks and live better lives.

However, following a gluten-free diet does not have to mean compromising flavor or diversity. With increased awareness of celiac illness, there are now several gluten-free options available, ranging from bread and pasta to snacks and sweets.

Accepting these alternatives may make the adjustment to a gluten-free diet easier and more pleasurable.

In short, controlling celiac disease requires rigorous adherence to a gluten-free diet. It's more than simply eliminating gluten; it's about regaining control of your health and well-being.

Dealing With Cross-Contamination

Cross-contamination is a major issue for celiac patients, since even small levels of gluten may cause a response. So, how do you negotiate this potential minefield?

First, it's critical to grasp what cross-contamination is. This happens when gluten-containing foods make contact with gluten-free meals, utensils, or surfaces, contaminating them. This may occur in communal kitchens, restaurants, or even at home if necessary measures are not taken.

To reduce the danger of cross-contamination, create a distinct gluten-free zone in your kitchen. This entails using different cutting boards, cutlery, and cooking equipment for gluten-free dishes. Furthermore, identifying gluten-free items and components might assist in avoiding confusion during meal preparation.

When eating out, communication is essential. Make sure to alert the restaurant staff about your dietary restrictions and inquire about their cross-contamination measures. Choosing restaurants with gluten-free menus or specialized gluten-free kitchens may also help to decrease the danger of inadvertent exposure.

Bringing your gluten-free foods to social situations, such as parties or gatherings, will assist guarantee that safe alternatives are accessible. Educating friends and family about celiac disease and the necessity of preventing cross-contamination may help to build understanding and support.

Finally, read labels carefully and keep knowledgeable about hidden gluten sources. Gluten-containing ingredients include modified food starch, malt vinegar, and hydrolyzed vegetable protein, so it's important to be aware of these possible culprits.

Individuals with celiac disease may get peace of mind and improved management of their illness by adopting proactive precautions to minimize cross-contamination.

Lifestyle Adjustments For Better Health

Managing celiac disease takes more than simply dietary modifications; it often necessitates making changes to different elements of everyday life to promote greater health and well-being.

One important lifestyle change is to prioritize self-care and stress management. Living with a chronic illness, such as celiac disease, may be stressful, particularly when dealing with social settings or eating out. Finding healthy ways to cope with stress, such as exercise, meditation, or hobbies, may assist to lessen its influence on overall health.

Furthermore, sufficient nutrition is critical for those with celiac disease since loss of nutrients may develop owing to intestinal injury. Working with a celiac disease specialist may assist you in developing a gluten-free diet that is both balanced and nutritionally adequate.

Regular exercise is an essential part of celiac disease management. It not only promotes general health and well-being, but it may also aid with symptoms like weariness and improving mood. Finding pleasurable kinds of physical activity, such as walking, cycling, or yoga, might help you keep to a consistent fitness schedule.

Having a strong support network is also advantageous for those with celiac disease. Connecting with individuals who understand the difficulties and successes of a gluten-free life may give motivation and useful information. Online networks, support groups, and advocacy organizations may provide direction, friendship, and a feeling of purpose.

Finally, remaining current on the newest research and breakthroughs in celiac disease care is critical. This involves being informed on gluten-free product alternatives, medical developments, and gluten-free lifestyle resources. Empowering yourself with information allows you to make educated choices and take charge of your health path.

Individuals with celiac disease may improve their health and well-being by implementing these lifestyle changes into their everyday lives, allowing them to live completely despite the limitations presented by their illness.

CHAPTER 6

Living With Celiac Disease

Coping Strategies For Emotional And Social Challenges

Living with celiac disease entails not only managing the medical components of the illness but also dealing with the emotional and social issues that accompany it. Coping skills may help you navigate these parts of everyday life.

Education is a good coping mechanism. Understanding the celiac disease, its symptoms, and the ramifications may help people make educated choices about their health and lifestyle. Individuals may recover control of their diet and lessen concern about accidental gluten exposure by learning about gluten-free options, checking food labels, and familiarizing themselves with safe dining techniques.

Communication is a key coping tool. Openly addressing celiac illness with friends, family, and colleagues may lead to greater understanding and support. Educating individuals close to you about the severity of the disease and the need to follow a rigorous gluten-free diet may help to avoid misconceptions and maintain a safe atmosphere in social situations.

Additionally, using mindfulness practices may help manage the stress associated with celiac disease. Meditation, deep breathing exercises, and yoga may all help people feel more grounded and less anxious. Mindfulness may also help identify and resolve negative thinking patterns associated with the disease, enhancing general mental health.

Participating in hobbies and activities that offer you pleasure and contentment may be helpful. Whether it's painting, gardening, or music, having avenues for creativity and self-expression may give a much-needed break from the difficulties of living with celiac disease. Investing time in hobbies may improve mood, resilience, and quality of life.

Finally, obtaining professional help when necessary is critical. Therapy or counseling may offer a secure environment in which to examine emotions, develop coping techniques, and treat any underlying psychological concerns associated with celiac disease. A mental health expert may provide counsel and support suited to an individual's requirements, promoting emotional healing and resilience.

Individuals with celiac disease who incorporate these coping methods into their everyday lives may better handle the emotional and social problems associated with the illness, resulting in increased overall well-being and quality of life.

Support Systems And Resources Available

Living with celiac disease necessitates access to support networks and tools to help negotiate the difficulties of maintaining a gluten-free diet. Fortunately, there are various services available to assist people to manage their disease properly.

Support groups are a wonderful resource. Connecting with individuals who have celiac disease may give you a feeling of belonging and understanding, which is essential for mental health. Support groups provide a forum for sharing stories, giving suggestions and information, and getting support from peers who understand the difficulties of living with the disease.

Individuals with celiac disease may also find a plethora of knowledge and support via online networks and forums. Platforms such as social media groups, specialized websites, and forums enable people to interact with others all over the globe, get up-to-date information about celiac disease, and seek assistance from professionals and other community members.

Furthermore, healthcare professionals play an important role in helping people with celiac disease. Consulting with a skilled healthcare team, which includes gastroenterologists, dietitians, and nutritionists, may help guarantee accurate diagnosis, management, and continuous support. These specialists can provide you with tailored advice on how to eat gluten-free, check your nutritional intake, and manage any celiac disease-related medical issues.

In addition to support groups and healthcare experts, there are several educational materials available to assist people learn more about celiac disease and gluten-free lifestyles. Books, blogs, podcasts, and instructional resources provide useful information about the disease, practical methods for managing it, and tasty gluten-free recipes to try at home.

Furthermore, many grocery shops and food manufacturers now provide gluten-free items, making it simpler than ever to locate safe and enjoyable alternatives for celiac disease patients. Online stores that specialize in gluten-free goods provide easy access to a diverse selection of products, such as pantry basics, snacks, and specialized items, enabling consumers to maintain a well-rounded gluten-free diet.

Individuals with celiac disease who use these support networks and services may successfully manage their illness, have access to essential information and assistance, and live happy lives while adhering to a gluten-free diet.

Thriving Beyond The Diagnosis

While getting a celiac disease diagnosis might be upsetting at first, it is possible to flourish thereafter with the correct attitude and support. Thriving with celiac disease entails accepting the illness as part of one's identity and making deliberate decisions to emphasize health and well-being.

Self-advocacy is an important part of living well with celiac disease. Advocating for one's requirements, whether that means conveying dietary limitations to restaurants or seeking gluten-free choices at social events, is critical for preserving health and avoiding gluten exposure. Individuals with celiac disease who articulate their demands boldly may guarantee that their dietary restrictions are respected and met in a variety of circumstances.

Furthermore, maintaining a good attitude is essential for living with celiac disease. Instead of perceiving the disease as a constraint, framing it as an opportunity for self-care and discovery may encourage people to embrace their gluten-free lifestyle with joy. Celebrating culinary ingenuity, finding new gluten-free dishes, and experimenting with alternative grains and ingredients may transform the gluten-free diet into a gourmet adventure rather than a constraint.

Building resilience is another critical component of living with celiac disease. Accepting the difficulties of the disease while also recognizing personal strengths and resources may help people build resilience in the face of adversity. Creating a support network of friends, family, and healthcare professionals may provide encouragement, insight, and practical aid on the path to flourishing with celiac disease.

Furthermore, emphasizing self-care and general well-being is critical for living with celiac disease. This involves engaging in regular exercise, prioritizing sleep, properly managing stress, and obtaining emotional assistance when necessary. Individuals with celiac disease may improve their overall quality of life and flourish by taking proactive actions to care for their physical and mental health.

To summarize, flourishing with celiac disease is feasible with the correct attitude, support, and resources. Individuals with celiac disease may live satisfying lives and reach their full potential by adopting self-advocacy, having a positive perspective, developing resilience, and emphasizing self-care.

CHAPTER 7

Gluten-Free Cooking And Recipes

Cooking Techniques And Ingredient Substitutions

Mastering gluten-free cooking entails learning different cooking methods and replacing products to make excellent gluten-free meals. Whether you're a novice or an experienced chef, these strategies and alternatives can help you improve your gluten-free cooking skills.

Cooking Techniques:

1. Grain Alternatives: Instead of wheat flour, use almond flour, coconut flour, rice flour, or chickpea flour. Each flour has a distinct taste profile and texture, so it's critical to choose the best match for your recipe.

2. Thickening Agents: Gluten-free alternatives to traditional thickeners, such as wheat flour, include cornstarch, arrowroot powder, and tapioca flour. These components complement sauces, gravies, and soups.

3. Baking Tip: When baking gluten-free, adding xanthan gum or guar gum to your flour mixture simulates the elasticity and structure that gluten gives. To obtain the ideal texture and flavor, try blending gluten-free flour.

4. Cross-contamination Awareness: To avoid cross-contamination, use separate utensils, cutting boards, and kitchen equipment for gluten-free cooking. Clean all surfaces carefully and double-check ingredient labels to verify they are gluten-free.

Ingredient substitutions:

1. **Flour Substitutes:** Replace wheat flour with gluten-free alternatives such as almond flour, coconut flour, or a flour mix. These alternatives have comparable binding qualities and may be used in most recipes with little changes.

2. **Breadcrumbs:** Crushed gluten-free crackers or gluten-free breadcrumbs may be used instead of typical breadcrumbs in dishes such as meatballs, breaded poultry, and stuffing.

3. **Soy Sauce Alternatives:** While traditional soy sauce includes wheat, gluten-free tamari or coconut aminos make good alternatives. They provide the same flavorful taste without the gluten.

4. **Pasta Swaps:** Enjoy pasta meals using gluten-free pasta made from rice, quinoa, or lentils.

These options cook similarly to wheat pasta and work well with a variety of sauces and toppings.

By learning these culinary methods and ingredient replacements, you can produce delectable gluten-free meals that everyone will love.

Delicious Gluten-Free Recipes For Every Meal

Transitioning to a gluten-free diet does not imply abandoning flavor or diversity. Discover these delectable gluten-free recipes for breakfast, lunch, supper, and snacks to keep your meals interesting and rewarding.

Breakfast: Gluten-free Banana Pancakes.

Begin the day properly with fluffy gluten-free banana pancakes. Mash ripe bananas and combine them with gluten-free flour, eggs, milk (or a dairy-free substitute), and a sprinkle of cinnamon. Cook the batter on a hot griddle until golden brown, then serve with fresh fruit and maple syrup for a delicious breakfast.

For a healthful and full lunch, try a quinoa salad with avocado, chickpeas, cherry tomatoes, and fresh herbs. Combine the ingredients with a zesty lemon vinaigrette prepared with olive oil, lemon juice, garlic, and Dijon mustard. This bright salad is loaded with protein, fiber, and taste.

Prepare a fast and delectable gluten-free chicken stir-fry for supper. Marinate chicken strips with gluten-free soy sauce, garlic, ginger, and sesame oil. Stir-fry the chicken with your favorite veggies, including bell peppers, broccoli, and snap peas, until soft. Serve with steamed rice or cauliflower rice for a full supper.

Snack: Homemade trail mix.

Keep hunger at bay by making your own gluten-free and personalized trail mix. In a large bowl, combine nuts, seeds, dried fruit, and gluten-free cereal. Mix thoroughly. Divide the trail mix into individual snack packs for easy on-the-go eating. Enjoy the crunchy, salty-sweet delight anytime you're hungry.

Tips For Meal Planning And Batch Cooking

Efficient meal planning and bulk cooking may make gluten-free eating easier and save time and effort on hectic weekdays. Follow these suggestions to simplify your meal planning and ensure you always have tasty gluten-free alternatives on hand.

Plan:

1. Create a Weekly Menu: At the start of each week, sit down and plan your meals, taking into consideration any gluten-free dishes you wish to try. Create a shopping list based on your menu to ensure you have all of the essential supplies.

2. Spend the day batch cooking gluten-free essentials such as quinoa, rice, roasted veggies, and grilled chicken. Store these goods in separate fridge or freezer containers to make it easier to construct meals throughout the week.

3. To expedite the cooking process, prepare items ahead of time by washing, chopping, and portioning them. Prepped veggies, cooked grains, and marinated meats may be refrigerated until ready to use.

Stay organized:

1. Label Containers: Keep track of what's in your fridge or freezer by clearly labeling containers with the date and contents.

This will allow you to prevent food waste and consume items before they expire.

2. Use Reusable Containers: Purchase a range of reusable containers in various sizes to keep prepared components and cooked meals. Choose glass containers with sealed closures for longevity and convenience.

3. Rotate Stock: When meal planning and batch cooking, move older products to the front of the fridge or freezer so they are consumed first. This reduces food waste and helps you keep your kitchen well-stocked.

By adopting these meal planning and batch cooking strategies into your daily routine, you can make gluten-free cooking easier and guarantee you always have great meals on hand.

CHAPTER 8

Navigating Social Situations

Explaining Celiac Disease To Family And Friends

When communicating celiac illness to your loved ones, clarity and patience are essential. Begin by informing them about celiac disease and how it affects the body. Explain that celiac disease is an autoimmune condition caused by the consumption of gluten, a protein found in wheat, barley, and rye. It damages the lining of the small intestine, resulting in a variety of symptoms and problems.

Describe the possible repercussions of ingesting gluten to demonstrate the severity of the illness, such as digestive problems, vitamin deficits, and long-term health difficulties.

Emphasize that the only way to cure celiac disease is to follow a rigorous gluten-free diet.

Provide practical examples to assist your family and friends in understanding which gluten-containing items to avoid and how to find gluten-free alternatives. Share personal experiences or tales to make the content more relevant and remembered.

Encourage open communication and welcome questions from loved ones. Assure them that their support and understanding are critical for good celiac disease management. Provide resources such as reliable websites or books for additional study, and try incorporating them in meal preparation or grocery shopping to build a feeling of community and collaboration.

Handling Social Events And Gatherings

Navigating social events and gatherings may be difficult for people with celiac disease, but with good planning and communication, it's completely achievable. Begin by researching the location or contacting the host to learn about gluten-free choices and accommodations.

If feasible, offer to bring a gluten-free food to share, ensuring you have a safe alternative to eat. Eating ahead of time or packing snacks might also help you avoid becoming hungry if gluten-free alternatives are limited.

Inform the host or organizer of your dietary preferences ahead of time, gently explaining your condition and any cross-contamination concerns. Provide instructions for safe food preparation procedures, such as using separate utensils and surfaces to avoid gluten contamination.

During the occasion, be alert and careful while choosing food products. Politely refuse gluten-containing foods and instead choose safer options.

Remember to firmly advocate for oneself while still being mindful of others' efforts and hospitality.

If other visitors express doubt or ignorance, politely restate the severity of celiac illness and the significance of avoiding gluten. Educate them on cross-contamination hazards and reassure them that your food restrictions are a medical necessity rather than a personal choice.

Advocating For Yourself In Various Settings

Advocating for oneself as a celiac disease patient requires aggressiveness, knowledge, and perseverance. Whether eating out, traveling, or attending medical appointments, it is critical to explain your demands clearly and convincingly.

When eating out, don't be afraid to ask questions regarding menu alternatives and food preparation techniques.

Request gluten-free meal changes or substitutes, and remind restaurant workers of the need for cross-contamination prevention.

When traveling, investigate gluten-free eating alternatives ahead of time and bring gluten-free snacks to ensure you have safe options on hand. Communicate your dietary preferences to airlines, hotels, and tour operators so that they can accommodate you throughout your travel.

During medical visits, speak up for yourself by actively engaging in talks about your treatment plan and voicing any concerns or questions you may have. Proactively seek recommendations from celiac disease experts or nutritionists.

Overall, speaking for oneself as someone with celiac disease requires confidence, boldness, and a desire to educate people about your illness. By taking proactive actions to convey your requirements and preferences, you may confidently navigate different settings while ensuring that your health and well-being are emphasized.

CHAPTER 9

Celiac Disease In Children

Recognizing Symptoms In Children

Recognizing celiac disease symptoms in children is critical for timely diagnosis and therapy. While symptoms may differ from kid to child, frequent indicators include diarrhea, constipation, stomach discomfort, and bloating. However, it is important to remember that not all children exhibit normal stomach symptoms. Instead, kids may endure weariness, irritation, delayed development, or even behavioral abnormalities.

As a parent or caregiver, you must be concerned about your child's health. Keep a look out for repeated or chronic symptoms, particularly after eating gluten-containing foods. If you suspect celiac disease based on your symptoms, you should visit a healthcare expert for an accurate examination and diagnosis. Remember that early identification may greatly enhance your child's quality of life and long-term health results.

Managing Celiac Disease In School Settings

To provide a safe and supportive environment for children with celiac disease, parents, healthcare professionals, and school personnel must work together. Communication is essential. Begin by alerting the school about your child's health and dietary requirements. This might include submitting a medical note or documents from your healthcare practitioner describing the required adjustments.

Work closely with the school cafeteria personnel to ensure they understand the need to minimize cross-contamination and offer gluten-free lunch alternatives. Educate teachers and other school workers about celiac disease, including symptoms and dietary restrictions, so they can better assist your kid in class.

Also, consider giving your kid a stockpile of gluten-free snacks or meals to keep at school in case of an emergency or unforeseen event. Encourage open communication between your kid and school professionals so that they feel free to share their needs and concerns.

Supporting Children With Celiac Disease

Supporting children with celiac disease involves more than simply regulating their food. It is critical to provide emotional support and enable them to advocate for their health care. Help your kid comprehend their illness by describing it in age-appropriate language and responding to any questions they may have.

Encourage your kid to take an active part in their nutrition by teaching them how to read product labels and identify gluten-containing substances. This may help children gain confidence in managing their disease, particularly as they age and become more independent.

Join support groups or online forums for celiac disease-affected families. Sharing experiences and advice with other parents and children may give useful information and comfort.

Finally, create a good and inclusive atmosphere at home and in social situations. Celebrate gluten-free options and emphasize the tasty things your kid can eat rather than the ones they must avoid. You may help your kid succeed despite celiac disease by building a support network and teaching them how to manage their illness.

CHAPTER 10

Future Perspectives And Research

Promising Advances In Celiac Disease Research

The future of celiac disease research seems promising, with continual breakthroughs targeted at better understanding the disorder, its causes, and possible therapies. Scientists and medical experts are diving deeper into the complex systems that underpin celiac disease, opening the path for novel diagnostic tools and therapeutics.

One of the most fascinating areas of study is identifying the genetic and immunological mechanisms that contribute to celiac disease. Researchers are gradually uncovering particular genetic markers connected with the illness, which provides insight into its hereditary origin.

This information not only assists in early diagnosis but also influences the creation of individualized treatment strategies based on an individual's genetic profile.

Furthermore, investigating the gut microbiota has emerged as a viable avenue in celiac disease research. Scientists are looking at how the mix of gut bacteria affects the disease's course. Understanding these intricate connections may lead to innovative treatment options, such as probiotic therapy that restores microbial balance while alleviating symptoms.

Another area of ongoing research is the creation of non-invasive diagnostic tools for celiac disease. While invasive treatments like gut biopsies are now the gold standard, researchers are looking into less stressful alternatives including blood-based testing and imaging tools. These developments not only improve the diagnostic process but also make it more accessible to patients, especially those who are hesitant to undergo invasive treatments.

Furthermore, there is rising interest in how environmental variables influence celiac disease initiation and progression. Researchers are investigating numerous environmental triggers, such as early-life nutritional exposures and viral infections, to better understand their influence on disease risk. Identifying these environmental variables allows us to develop disease preventive and treatment measures, eventually improving patient outcomes.

In summary, the future of celiac disease research is defined by multidisciplinary cooperation and innovation, with the ultimate objective of increasing diagnostic accuracy, creating targeted therapeutics, and improving the quality of life for those living with an autoimmune disorder.

Potential Therapies And Treatments On The Horizon

The landscape of celiac disease medicines and treatments is changing, giving hope to those struggling with gluten sensitivity. While rigorous adherence to a gluten-free diet remains the cornerstone of care, researchers are looking into new methods to alleviate symptoms and target the underlying immunological response.

One of the most promising areas of research is the development of pharmacological medicines that control the immune system's abnormal reaction to gluten. These therapies seek to give comfort to celiac disease patients by enabling them to ingest gluten-containing foods without causing harmful inflammation in the small intestine.

One way is to employ enzyme supplements that may degrade gluten molecules in the digestive system, lowering their immunogenicity. While still in the early stage, these enzyme-based therapeutics show promise in minimizing the effects of accidental gluten intake and lowering dietary restrictions for celiac patients.

In addition to pharmacological therapies, researchers are investigating the viability of immunomodulatory medications that target particular immune system components involved in celiac disease development. By modifying immunological responses, these innovative medicines aim to reduce inflammation and prevent tissue damage caused by gluten consumption.

Furthermore, breakthroughs in science have made it possible to produce gluten-detoxifying agents capable of making gluten-containing foods safe for celiac disease patients to consume. These novel chemicals, which may include enzymes or binding agents, show potential as supplementary therapy for gluten-free diets and improve general quality of life.

In addition to pharmaceutical methods, researchers are exploring the possibility of immunotherapy as a long-term management strategy for celiac disease. Immunotherapy is progressively exposing patients to modest, controlled amounts of gluten to desensitize the immune system and develop tolerance. While still in the preliminary phases, immunotherapy has the potential to be a transforming therapeutic option for those who are limited by their gluten-free diet.

The landscape of celiac disease therapies and treatments is rapidly changing, with promising developments on the horizon. From enzyme supplements to immunomodulatory drugs and immunotherapy, these novel approaches provide hope for better symptom management and a higher quality of life for celiac patients.

Advocacy And Awareness Efforts For Celiac Disease

Advocacy and awareness initiatives are critical in increasing awareness and understanding of celiac disease, fostering support for affected individuals, and driving advancements in research and healthcare. Advocates work tirelessly to raise the voices of those affected by the condition, promoting inclusivity, accessibility, and equitable treatment for all.

The dissemination of accurate information about celiac disease, including symptoms, diagnosis, and treatment, is critical to advocacy efforts. By raising awareness among healthcare providers, policymakers, and the general public, advocates hope to facilitate timely diagnosis, improve access to gluten-free options, and foster a supportive environment for people living with celiac disease.

Furthermore, advocacy organizations play an important role in advocating for policy changes that protect the rights and well-being of people living with celiac disease. These efforts, which range from advocating for clear labeling of gluten-containing products to promoting gluten-free accommodations in schools, workplaces, and public spaces, seek to remove barriers and promote inclusivity for those who follow gluten-free diets.

In addition to policy advocacy, awareness campaigns are effective at dispelling myths and misconceptions about celiac disease. Advocates empower people with celiac disease by sharing personal stories, educational resources, and practical gluten-free living tips.

Furthermore, advocacy efforts go beyond traditional awareness campaigns and include community building and support networks. Individuals suffering from celiac disease can find solidarity, camaraderie, and invaluable resources for dealing with the physical, emotional, and social aspects of their condition through support groups, online forums, and social media platforms.

In essence, advocacy and awareness efforts help to drive positive change and improve outcomes for people suffering from celiac disease. Advocates pave the way for greater understanding, acceptance, and support for those dealing with gluten intolerance by amplifying voices, eradicating stigma, and fostering community.

CONCLUSION

In conclusion, Celiac Disease is a complex autoimmune disorder caused by the body's reaction to gluten, a protein found in wheat, barley, and rye. If left untreated, this condition can have a significant impact on an individual's quality of life. Several key points have emerged during this discussion about the diagnosis, treatment, and management of Celiac Disease.

For starters, individuals suspected of having Celiac Disease must receive an accurate diagnosis. Blood tests to detect specific antibodies are typically used in conjunction with small intestine biopsies to confirm the diagnosis. Early detection enables timely intervention and lowers the risk of long-term complications associated with untreated celiac disease.

Second, strict adherence to a gluten-free diet is essential for effective management. Eliminating gluten-containing foods is critical for relieving symptoms, promoting intestinal healing, and preventing further damage to the small bowel. However, because gluten is commonly found in many food products, adhering to a gluten-free diet can be difficult. Individuals with Celiac disease require ongoing education and support from healthcare professionals, dietitians, and support groups.

Additionally, it is critical to address any nutritional deficiencies caused by malabsorption in the small intestine. Supplementation with vitamins and minerals, particularly iron, calcium, and vitamin D, may be required to restore optimal health.

Furthermore, ongoing monitoring is required to evaluate treatment efficacy, ensure nutritional adequacy, and detect any potential complications or associated conditions, such as dermatitis herpetiformis or osteoporosis.

To summarize, while living with Celiac Disease necessitates significant dietary changes and vigilance, people can live healthy and fulfilling lives with proper treatment. By increasing awareness, improving diagnostic methods, and providing support systems, we can help people with Celiac Disease navigate the challenges of their condition and improve their overall well-being.

THE END